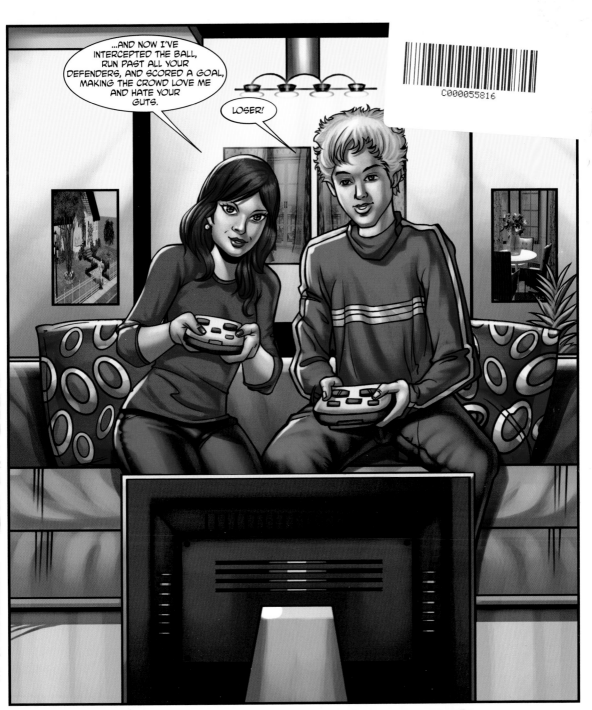

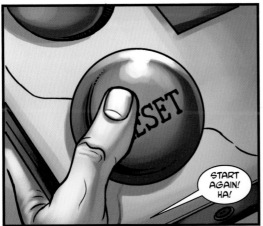

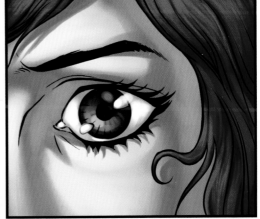

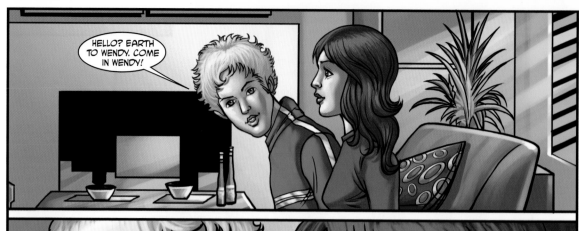

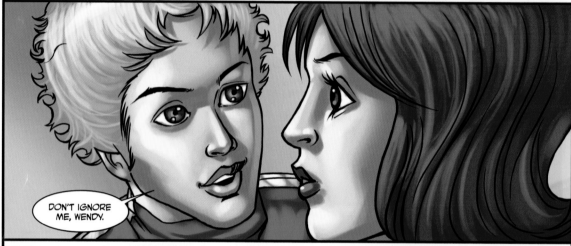

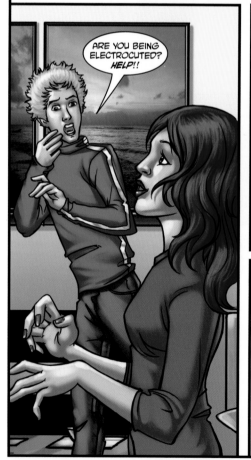

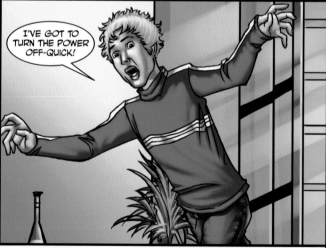

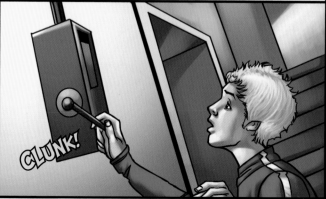

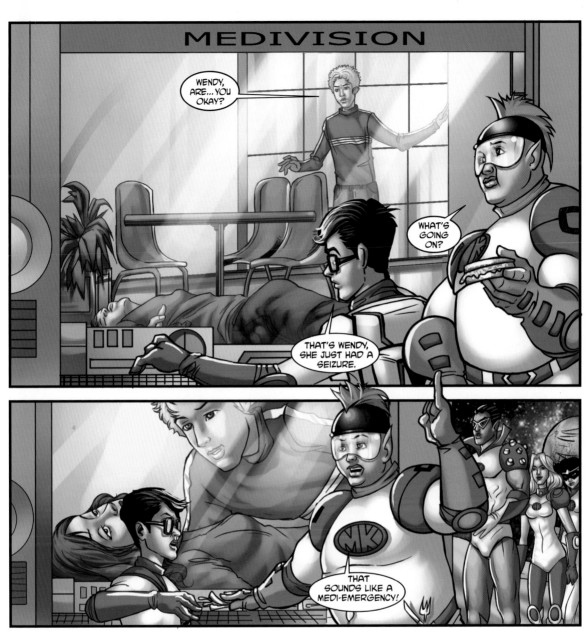

WENDY, ARE...YOU OKAY?

WHAT'S GOING ON?

THAT'S WENDY, SHE JUST HAD A SEIZURE.

THAT SOUNDS LIKE A MEDI-EMERGENCY!

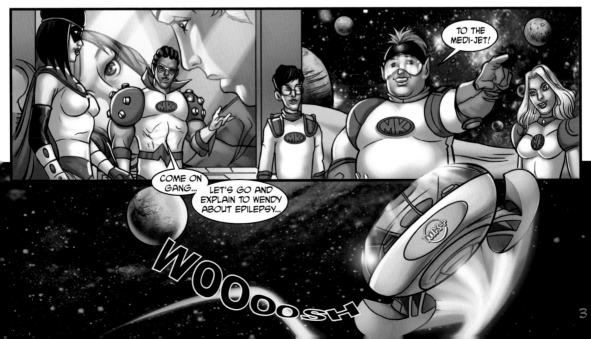

TO THE MEDI-JET!

COME ON GANG... LET'S GO AND EXPLAIN TO WENDY ABOUT EPILEPSY...

WOOOOSH

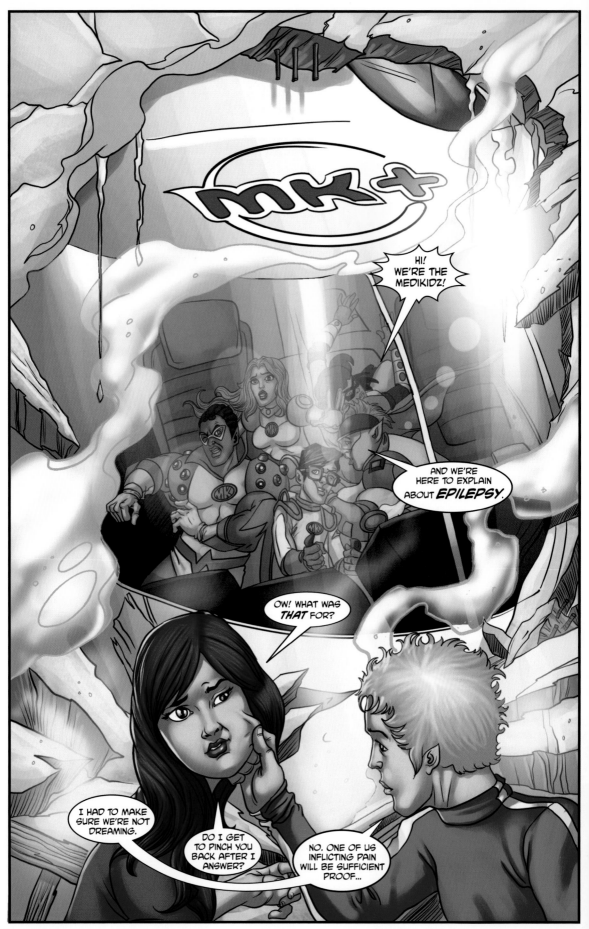

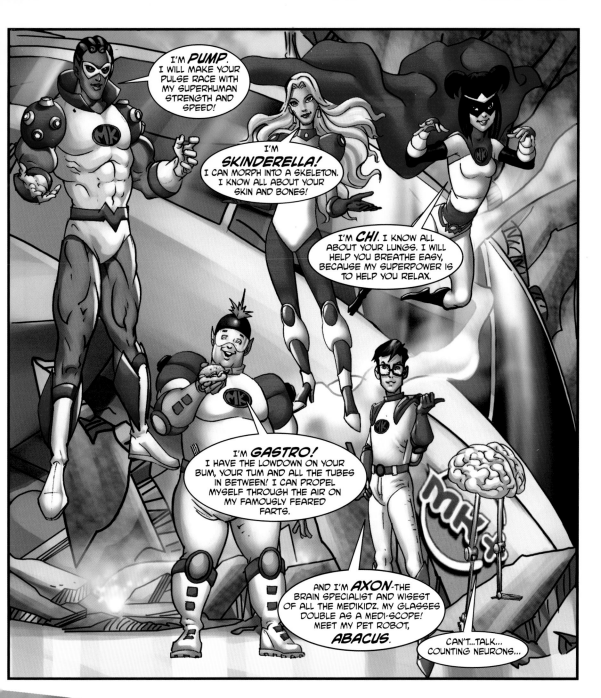

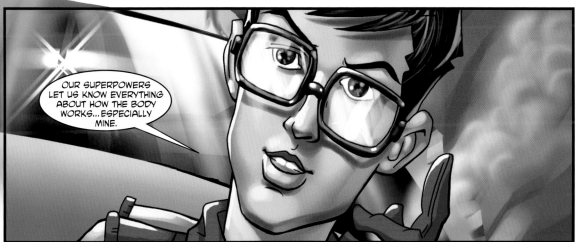

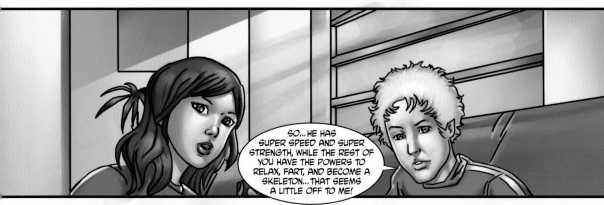

SO...HE HAS SUPER SPEED AND SUPER STRENGTH, WHILE THE REST OF YOU HAVE THE POWERS TO RELAX, FART, AND BECOME A SKELETON...THAT SEEMS A LITTLE OFF TO ME!

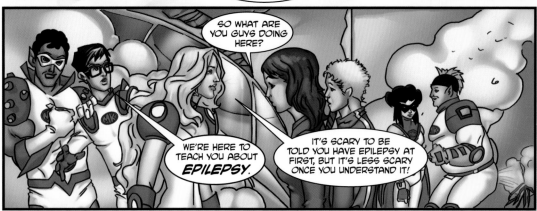

SO WHAT ARE YOU GUYS DOING HERE?

WE'RE HERE TO TEACH YOU ABOUT *EPILEPSY*.

IT'S SCARY TO BE TOLD YOU HAVE EPILEPSY AT FIRST, BUT IT'S LESS SCARY ONCE YOU UNDERSTAND IT!

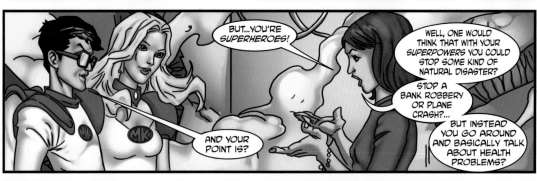

BUT...YOU'RE SUPERHEROES!

WELL, ONE WOULD THINK THAT WITH YOUR SUPERPOWERS YOU COULD STOP SOME KIND OF NATURAL DISASTER?

AND YOUR POINT IS?

STOP A BANK ROBBERY OR PLANE CRASH?...

BUT INSTEAD YOU GO AROUND AND BASICALLY TALK ABOUT HEALTH PROBLEMS?

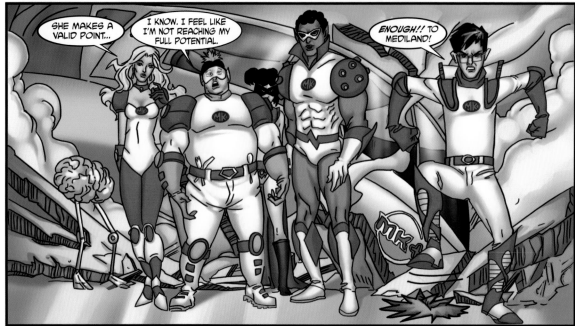

SHE MAKES A VALID POINT...

I KNOW. I FEEL LIKE I'M NOT REACHING MY FULL POTENTIAL.

ENOUGH!! TO MEDILAND!

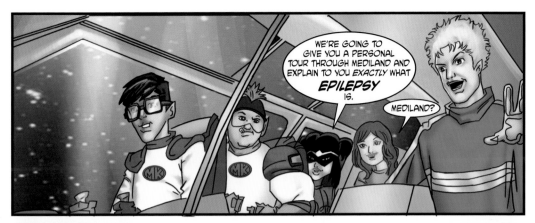

WE'RE GOING TO GIVE YOU A PERSONAL TOUR THROUGH MEDILAND AND EXPLAIN TO YOU *EXACTLY* WHAT **EPILEPSY** IS.

MEDILAND?

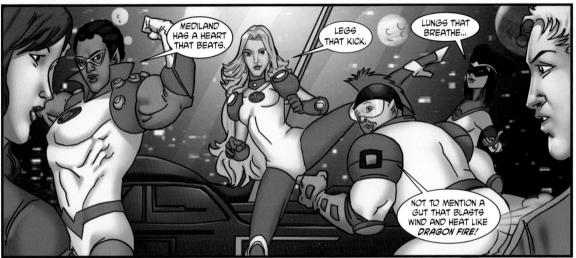

MEDILAND HAS A HEART THAT BEATS.

LEGS THAT KICK.

LUNGS THAT BREATHE...

NOT TO MENTION A GUT THAT BLASTS WIND AND HEAT LIKE *DRAGON FIRE!*

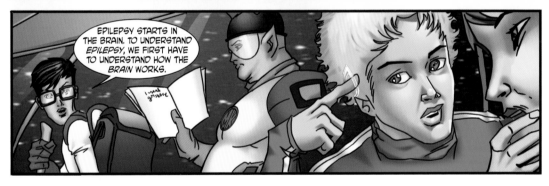

EPILEPSY STARTS IN THE BRAIN. TO UNDERSTAND *EPILEPSY*, WE FIRST HAVE TO UNDERSTAND HOW THE *BRAIN* WORKS.

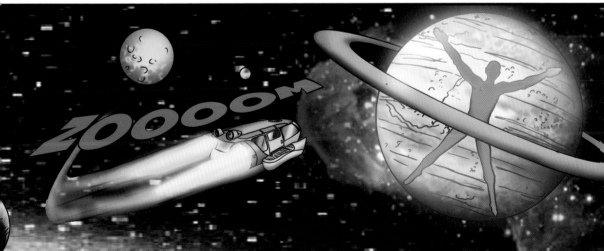

ZOOOOM

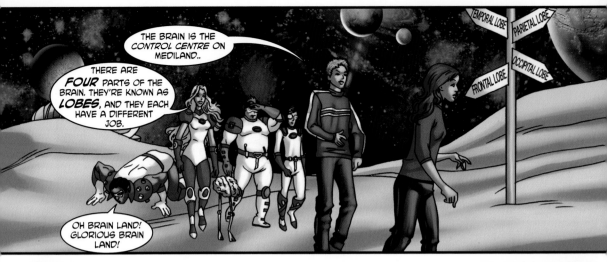

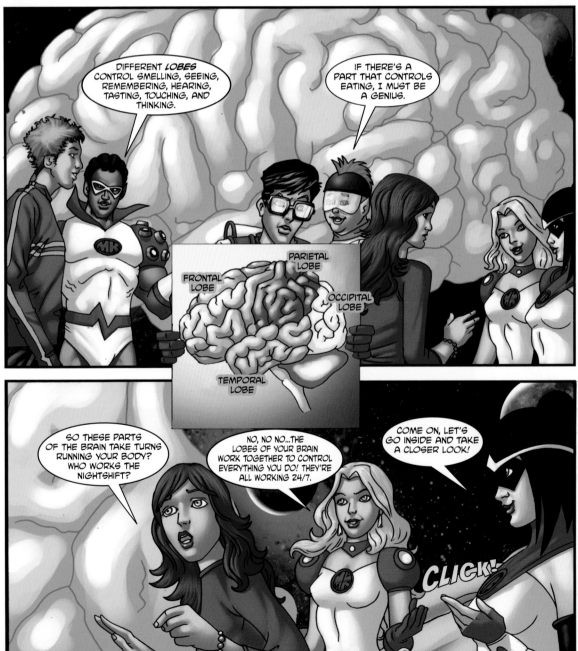

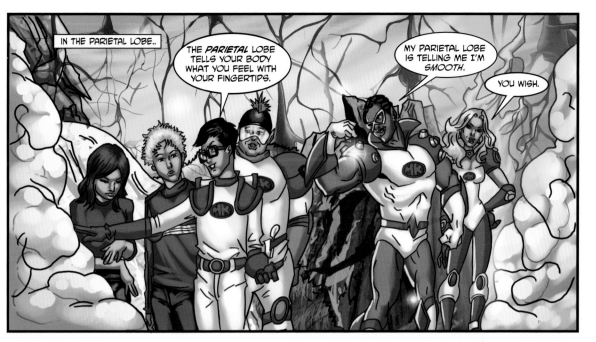

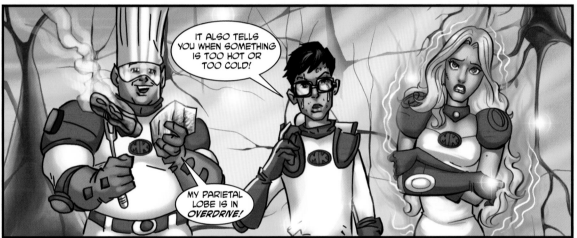

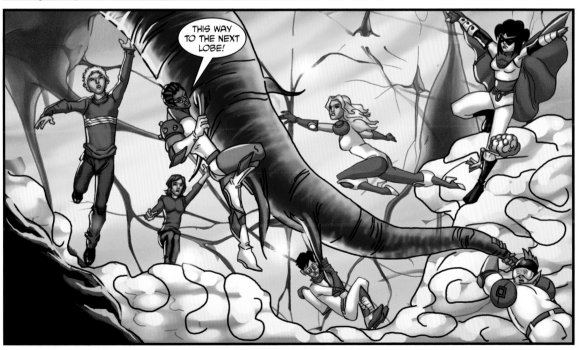

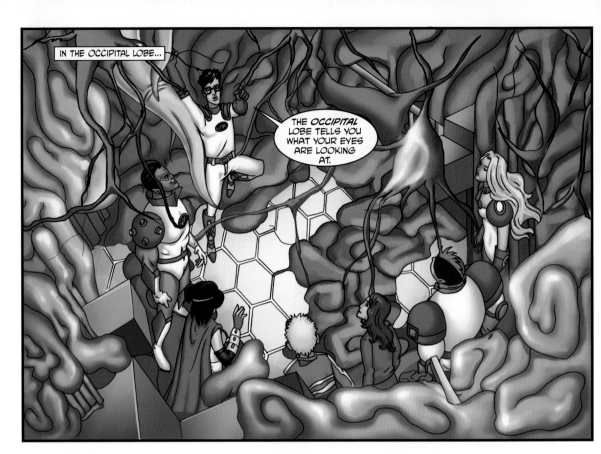

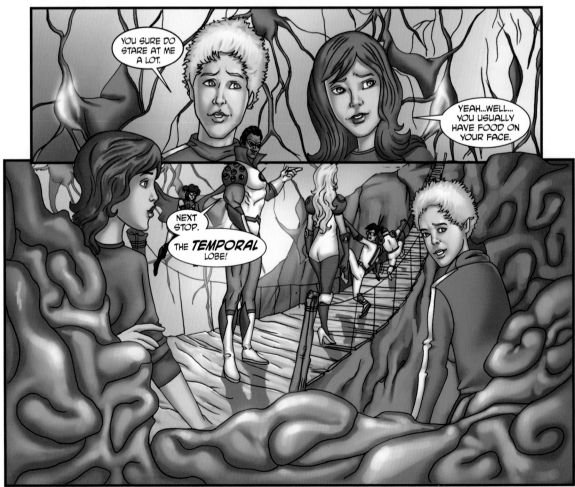

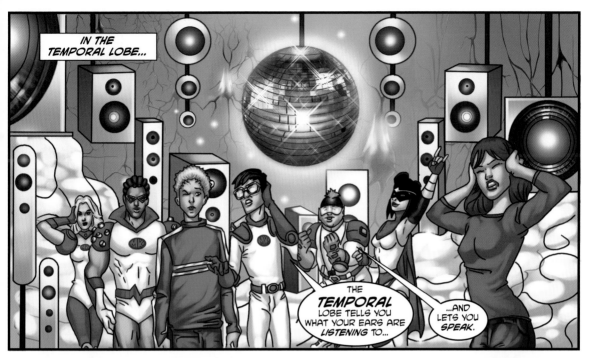

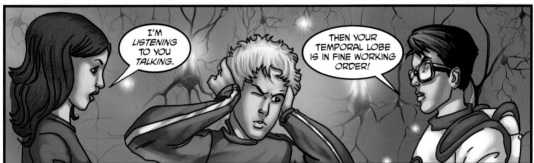

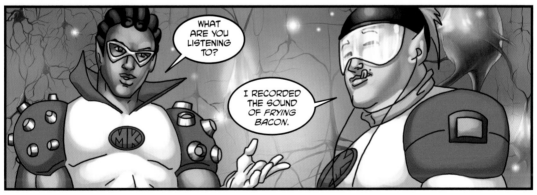

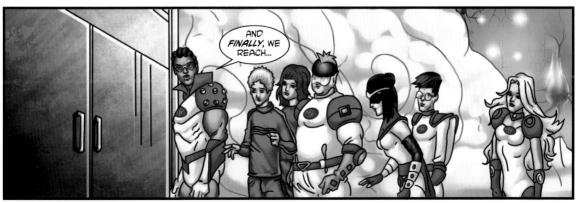

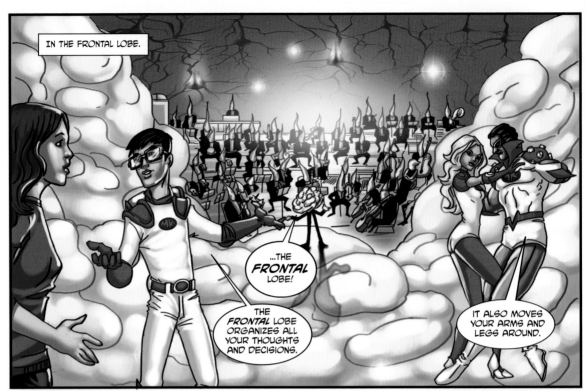

IN THE FRONTAL LOBE.

...THE *FRONTAL* LOBE!

THE *FRONTAL* LOBE ORGANIZES ALL YOUR THOUGHTS AND DECISIONS.

IT ALSO MOVES YOUR ARMS AND LEGS AROUND.

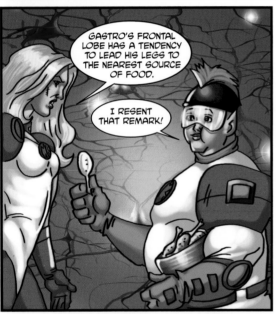

GASTRO'S FRONTAL LOBE HAS A TENDENCY TO LEAD HIS LEGS TO THE NEAREST SOURCE OF FOOD.

I RESENT THAT REMARK!

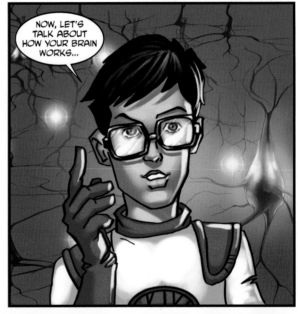

NOW, LET'S TALK ABOUT HOW YOUR BRAIN WORKS...

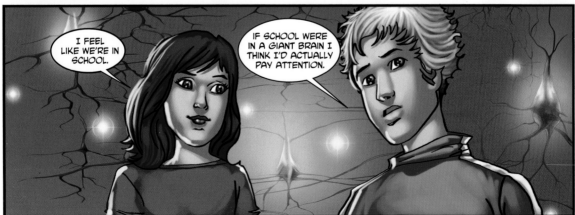

I FEEL LIKE WE'RE IN SCHOOL.

IF SCHOOL WERE IN A GIANT BRAIN I THINK I'D ACTUALLY PAY ATTENTION.

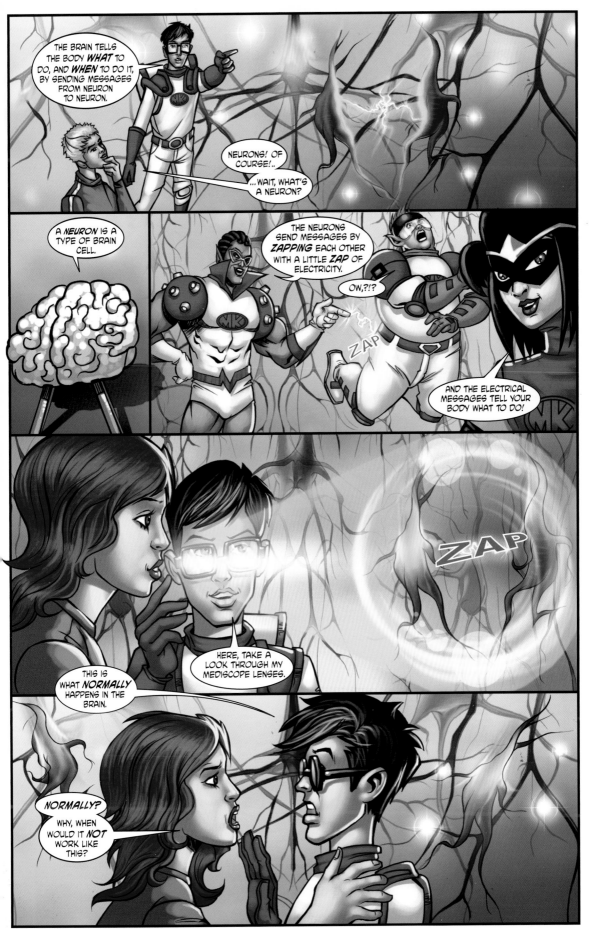

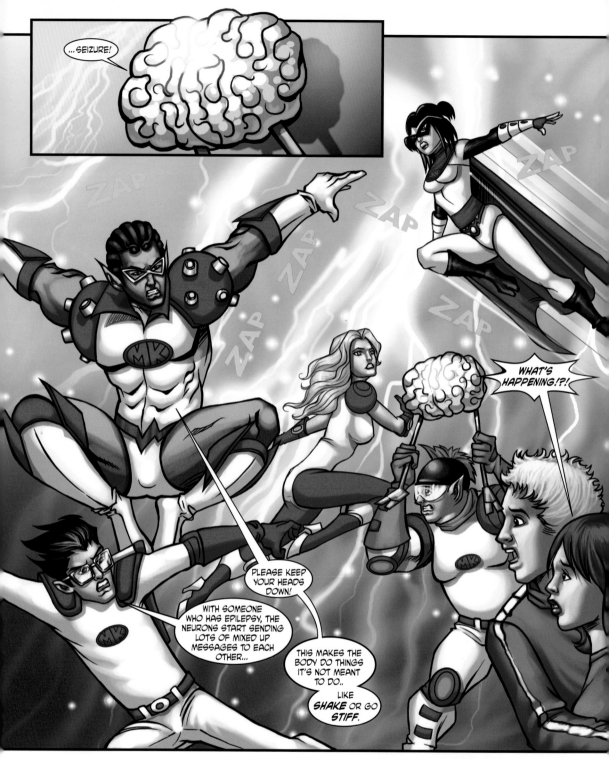

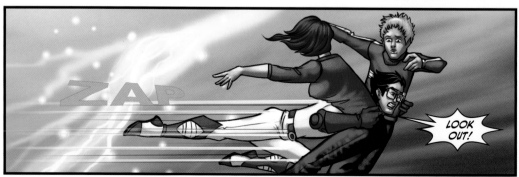

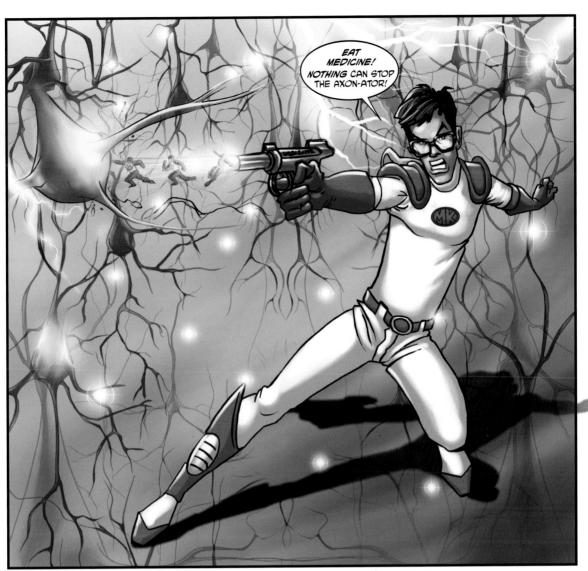

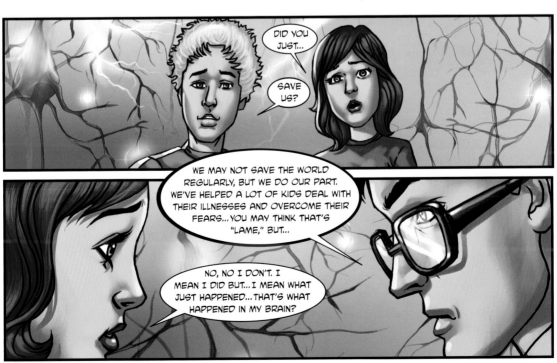

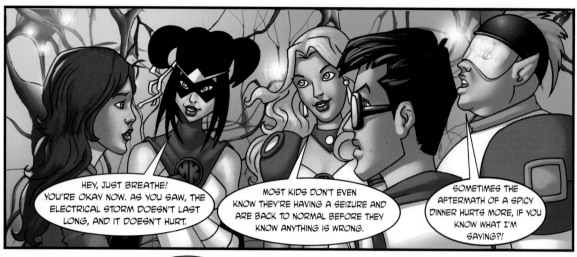

HEY, JUST BREATHE! YOU'RE OKAY NOW. AS YOU SAW, THE ELECTRICAL STORM DOESN'T LAST LONG, AND IT DOESN'T HURT.

MOST KIDS DON'T EVEN KNOW THEY'RE HAVING A SEIZURE AND ARE BACK TO NORMAL BEFORE THEY KNOW ANYTHING IS WRONG.

SOMETIMES THE AFTERMATH OF A SPICY DINNER HURTS MORE, IF YOU KNOW WHAT I'M SAYING?!

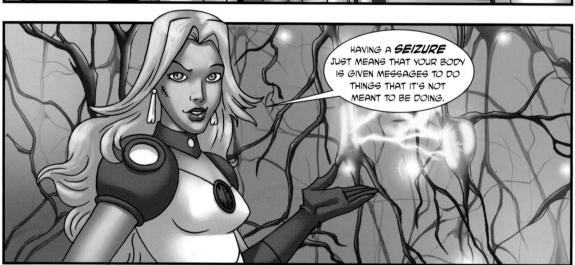

HAVING A *SEIZURE* JUST MEANS THAT YOUR BODY IS GIVEN MESSAGES TO DO THINGS THAT IT'S NOT MEANT TO BE DOING.

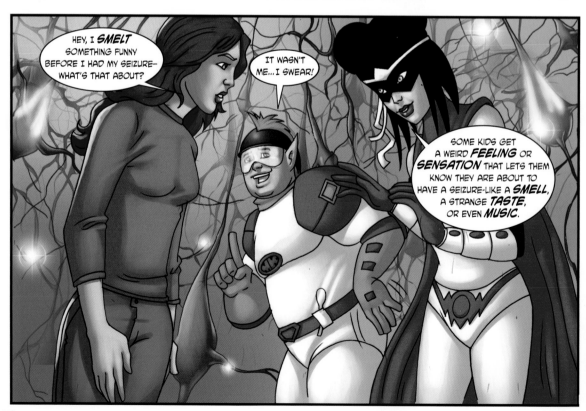

HEY, I *SMELT* SOMETHING FUNNY BEFORE I HAD MY SEIZURE— WHAT'S THAT ABOUT?

IT WASN'T ME... I SWEAR!

SOME KIDS GET A WEIRD *FEELING* OR *SENSATION* THAT LETS THEM KNOW THEY ARE ABOUT TO HAVE A SEIZURE-LIKE A *SMELL*, A STRANGE *TASTE*, OR EVEN *MUSIC*.

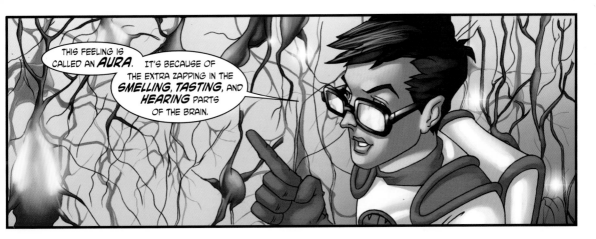

THIS FEELING IS CALLED AN **AURA**. IT'S BECAUSE OF THE EXTRA ZAPPING IN THE **SMELLING, TASTING,** AND **HEARING** PARTS OF THE BRAIN.

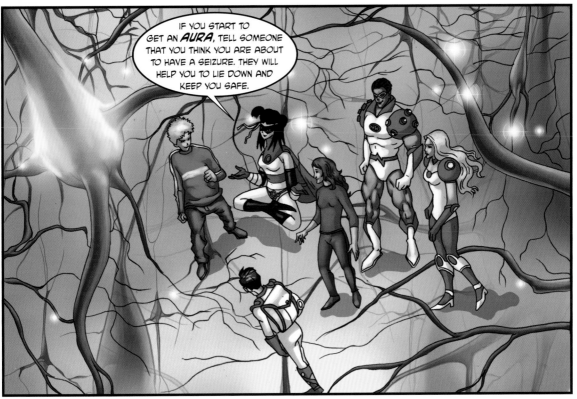

IF YOU START TO GET AN **AURA**, TELL SOMEONE THAT YOU THINK YOU ARE ABOUT TO HAVE A SEIZURE. THEY WILL HELP YOU TO LIE DOWN AND KEEP YOU SAFE.

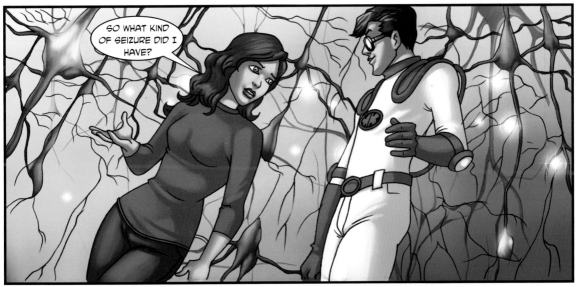

SO WHAT KIND OF SEIZURE DID I HAVE?

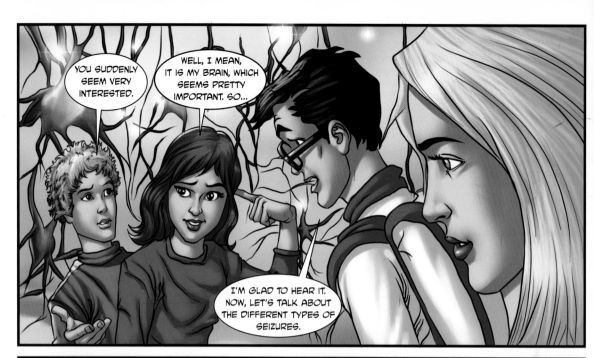

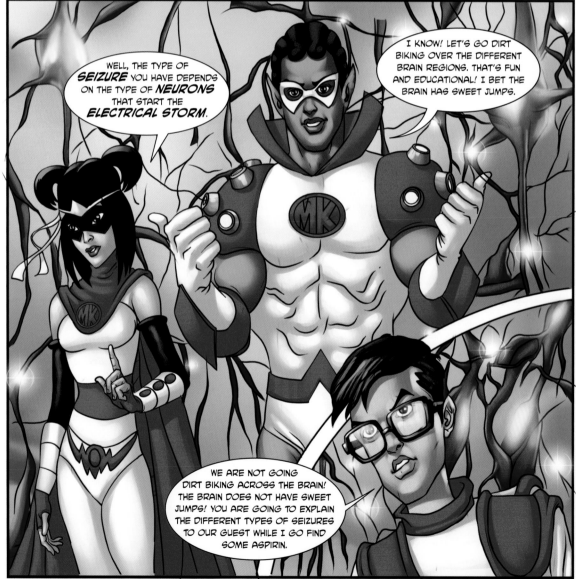

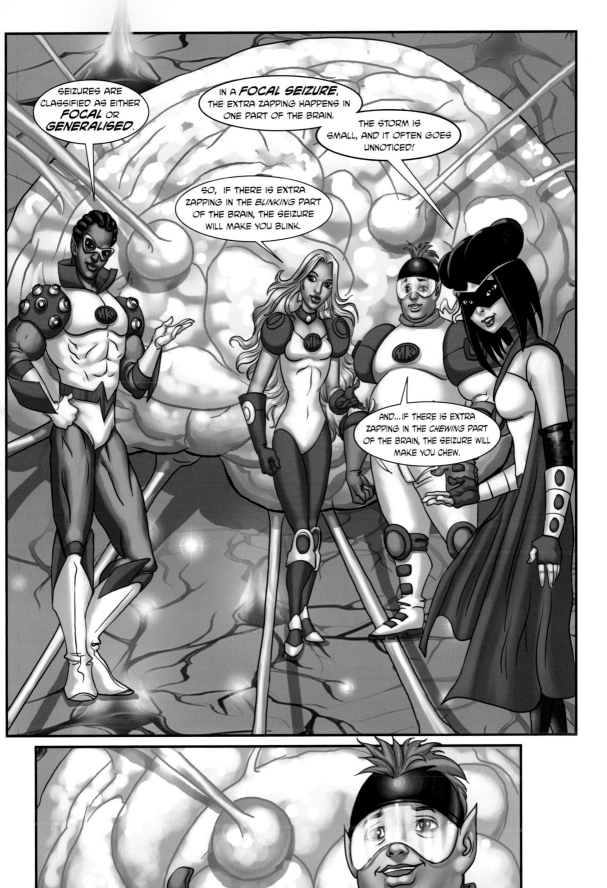

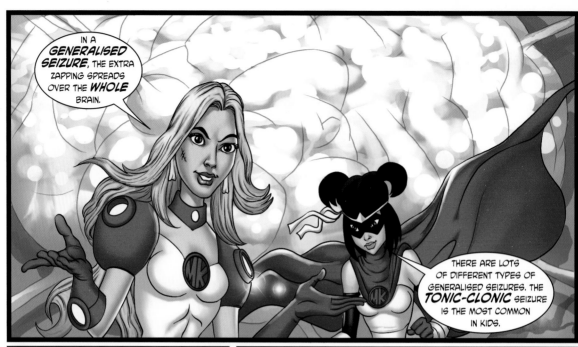

IN A **GENERALISED SEIZURE**, THE EXTRA ZAPPING SPREADS OVER THE **WHOLE** BRAIN.

THERE ARE LOTS OF DIFFERENT TYPES OF GENERALISED SEIZURES. THE **TONIC-CLONIC** SEIZURE IS THE MOST COMMON IN KIDS.

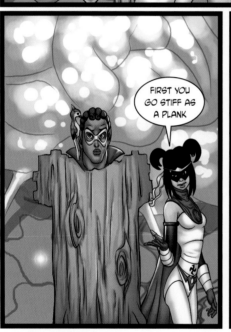

FIRST YOU GO STIFF AS A PLANK

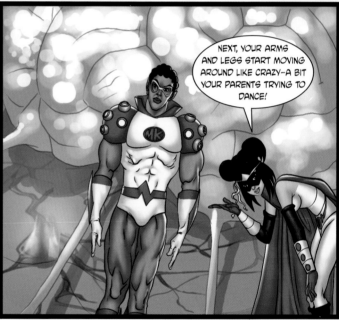

NEXT, YOUR ARMS AND LEGS START MOVING AROUND LIKE CRAZY-A BIT YOUR PARENTS TRYING TO DANCE!

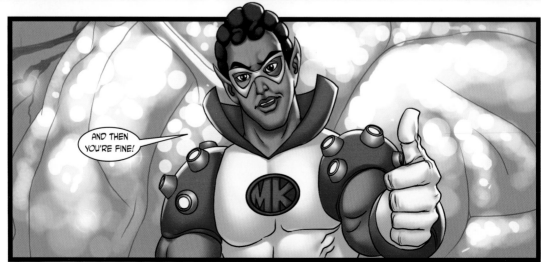

AND THEN YOU'RE FINE!

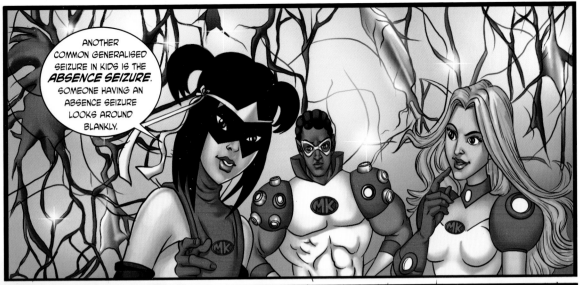

ANOTHER COMMON GENERALISED SEIZURE IN KIDS IS THE **ABSENCE SEIZURE**. SOMEONE HAVING AN ABSENCE SEIZURE LOOKS AROUND BLANKLY.

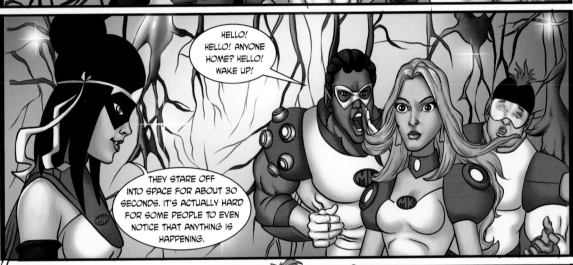

HELLO! HELLO! ANYONE HOME? HELLO! WAKE UP!

THEY STARE OFF INTO SPACE FOR ABOUT 30 SECONDS. IT'S ACTUALLY HARD FOR SOME PEOPLE TO EVEN NOTICE THAT ANYTHING IS HAPPENING.

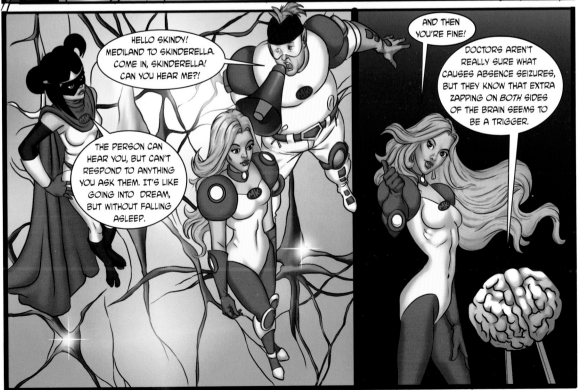

HELLO SKINDY! MEDILAND TO SKINDERELLA. COME IN, SKINDERELLA! CAN YOU HEAR ME?!

THE PERSON CAN HEAR YOU, BUT CAN'T RESPOND TO ANYTHING YOU ASK THEM. IT'S LIKE GOING INTO DREAM, BUT WITHOUT FALLING ASLEEP.

AND THEN YOU'RE FINE!

DOCTORS AREN'T REALLY SURE WHAT CAUSES ABSENCE SEIZURES, BUT THEY KNOW THAT EXTRA ZAPPING ON *BOTH* SIDES OF THE BRAIN SEEMS TO BE A TRIGGER.

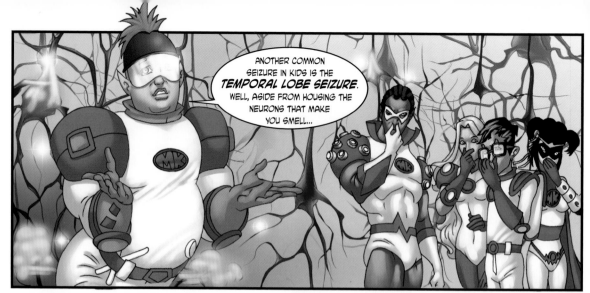

ANOTHER COMMON SEIZURE IN KIDS IS THE **TEMPORAL LOBE SEIZURE**. WELL, ASIDE FROM HOUSING THE NEURONS THAT MAKE YOU SMELL...

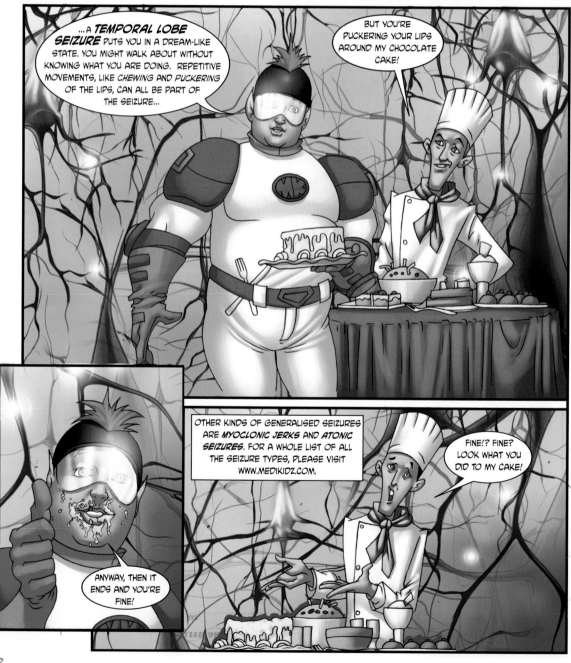

...A **TEMPORAL LOBE SEIZURE** PUTS YOU IN A DREAM-LIKE STATE. YOU MIGHT WALK ABOUT WITHOUT KNOWING WHAT YOU ARE DOING. REPETITIVE MOVEMENTS, LIKE *CHEWING* AND *PUCKERING* OF THE LIPS, CAN ALL BE PART OF THE SEIZURE...

BUT YOU'RE PUCKERING YOUR LIPS AROUND MY CHOCOLATE CAKE!

ANYWAY, THEN IT ENDS AND YOU'RE FINE!

OTHER KINDS OF GENERALISED SEIZURES ARE *MYOCLONIC JERKS* AND *ATONIC SEIZURES*. FOR A WHOLE LIST OF ALL THE SEIZURE TYPES, PLEASE VISIT WWW.MEDIKIDZ.COM.

FINE!? FINE? LOOK WHAT YOU DID TO MY CAKE!

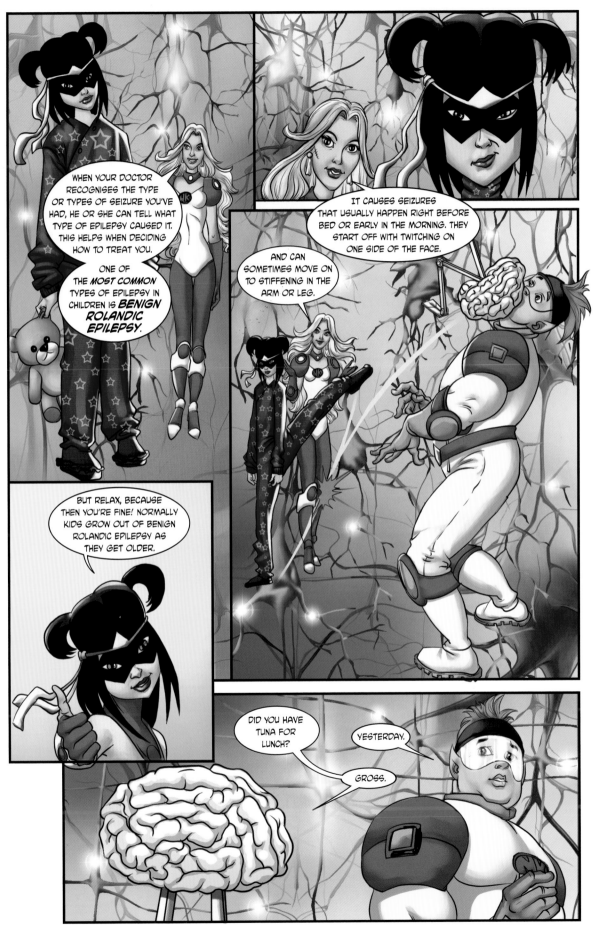

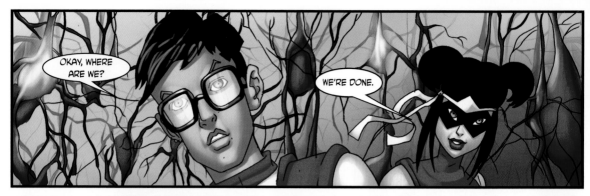

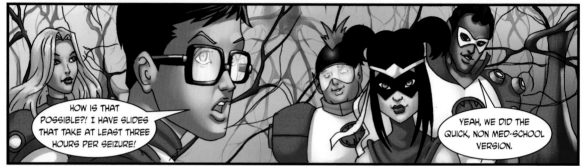

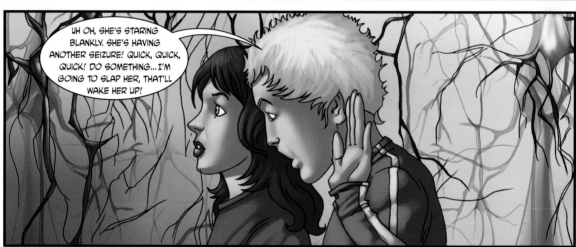

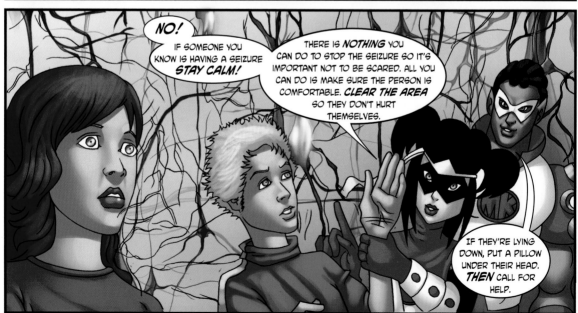

24

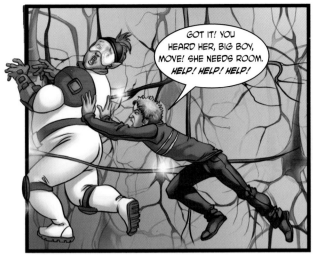

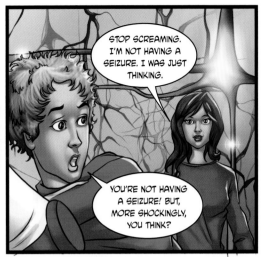

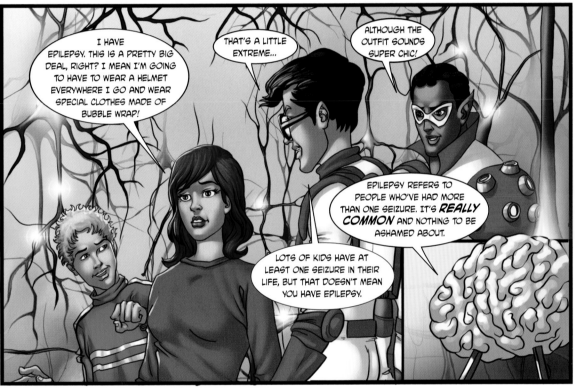

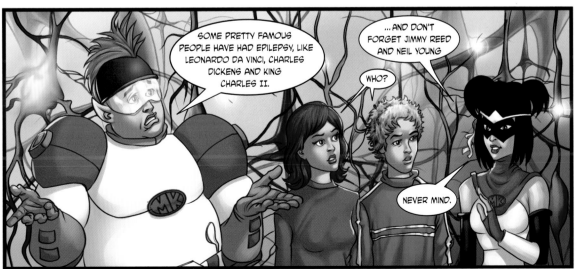

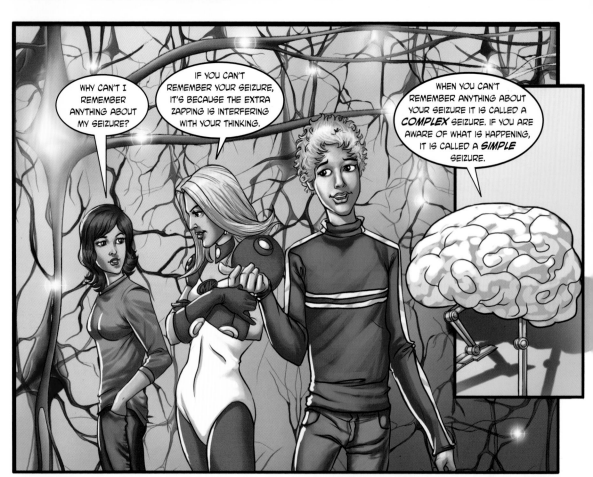

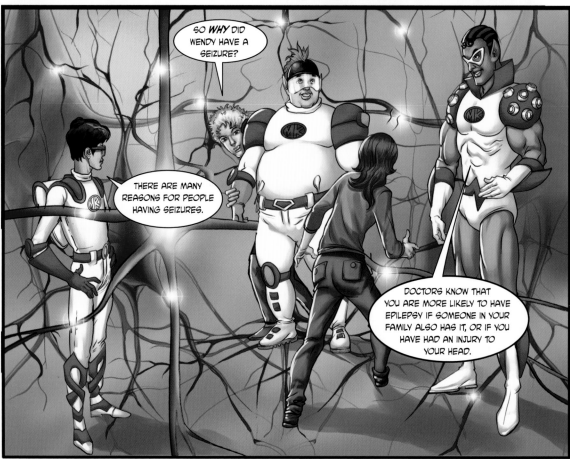

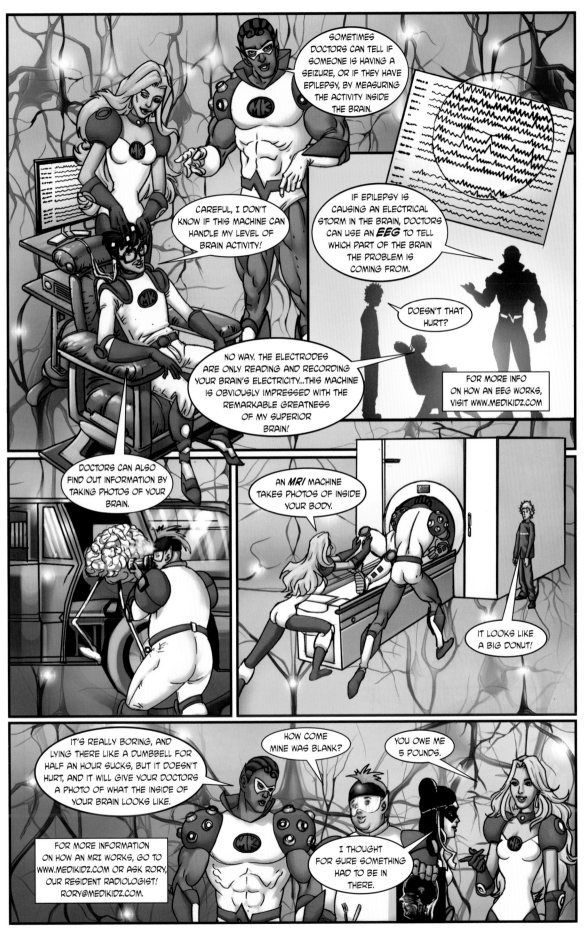

SOMETIMES DOCTORS CAN TELL IF SOMEONE IS HAVING A SEIZURE, OR IF THEY HAVE EPILEPSY, BY MEASURING THE ACTIVITY INSIDE THE BRAIN.

CAREFUL, I DON'T KNOW IF THIS MACHINE CAN HANDLE MY LEVEL OF BRAIN ACTIVITY!

IF EPILEPSY IS CAUSING AN ELECTRICAL STORM IN THE BRAIN, DOCTORS CAN USE AN *EEG* TO TELL WHICH PART OF THE BRAIN THE PROBLEM IS COMING FROM.

DOESN'T THAT HURT?

NO WAY. THE ELECTRODES ARE ONLY READING AND RECORDING YOUR BRAIN'S ELECTRICITY...THIS MACHINE IS OBVIOUSLY IMPRESSED WITH THE REMARKABLE GREATNESS OF MY SUPERIOR BRAIN!

FOR MORE INFO ON HOW AN EEG WORKS, VISIT WWW.MEDIKIDZ.COM

DOCTORS CAN ALSO FIND OUT INFORMATION BY TAKING PHOTOS OF YOUR BRAIN.

AN *MRI* MACHINE TAKES PHOTOS OF INSIDE YOUR BODY.

IT LOOKS LIKE A BIG DONUT!

IT'S REALLY BORING, AND LYING THERE LIKE A DUMBBELL FOR HALF AN HOUR SUCKS, BUT IT DOESN'T HURT, AND IT WILL GIVE YOUR DOCTORS A PHOTO OF WHAT THE INSIDE OF YOUR BRAIN LOOKS LIKE.

HOW COME MINE WAS BLANK?

YOU OWE ME 5 POUNDS.

FOR MORE INFORMATION ON HOW AN MRI WORKS, GO TO WWW.MEDIKIDZ.COM OR ASK RORY, OUR RESIDENT RADIOLOGIST! RORY@MEDIKIDZ.COM.

I THOUGHT FOR SURE SOMETHING HAD TO BE IN THERE.

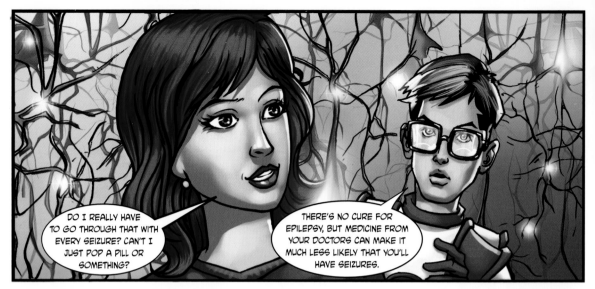

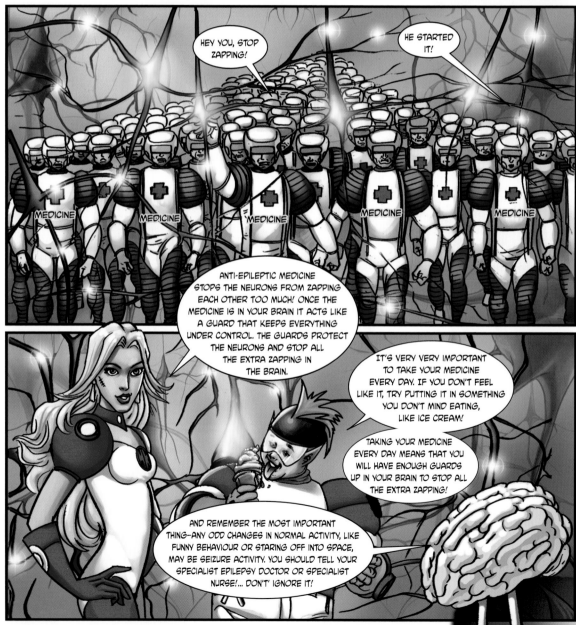

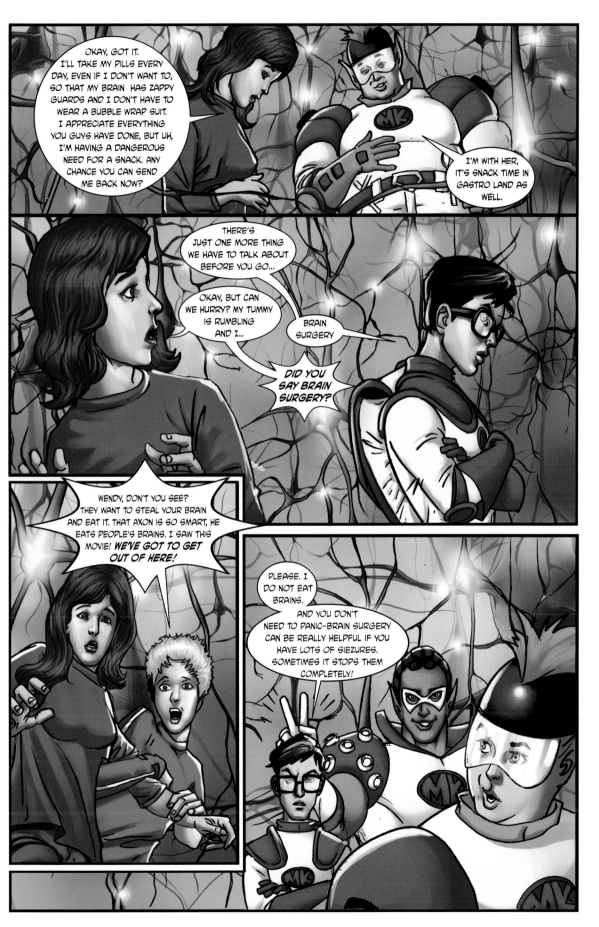

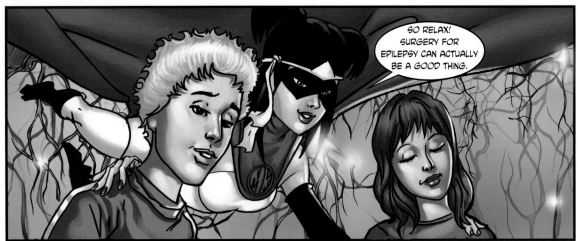

SO RELAX! SURGERY FOR EPILEPSY CAN ACTUALLY BE A GOOD THING.

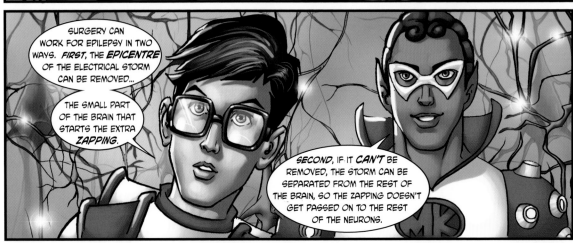

SURGERY CAN WORK FOR EPILEPSY IN TWO WAYS. *FIRST*, THE *EPICENTRE* OF THE ELECTRICAL STORM CAN BE REMOVED...

THE SMALL PART OF THE BRAIN THAT STARTS THE EXTRA *ZAPPING.*

SECOND, IF IT *CAN'T* BE REMOVED, THE STORM CAN BE SEPARATED FROM THE REST OF THE BRAIN, SO THE ZAPPING DOESN'T GET PASSED ON TO THE REST OF THE NEURONS.

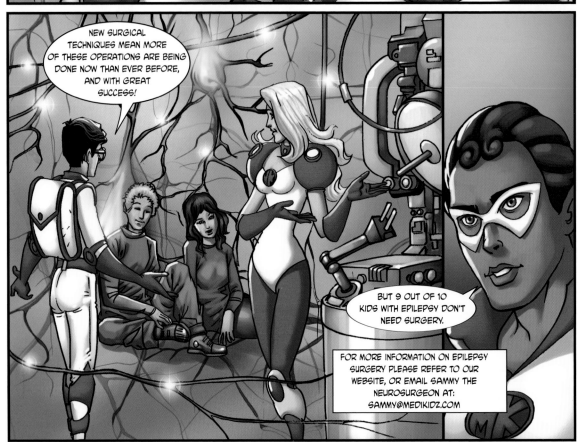

NEW SURGICAL TECHNIQUES MEAN MORE OF THESE OPERATIONS ARE BEING DONE NOW THAN EVER BEFORE, AND WITH GREAT SUCCESS!

BUT 9 OUT OF 10 KIDS WITH EPILEPSY DON'T NEED SURGERY.

FOR MORE INFORMATION ON EPILEPSY SURGERY PLEASE REFER TO OUR WEBSITE, OR EMAIL SAMMY THE NEUROSURGEON AT: SAMMY@MEDIKIDZ.COM

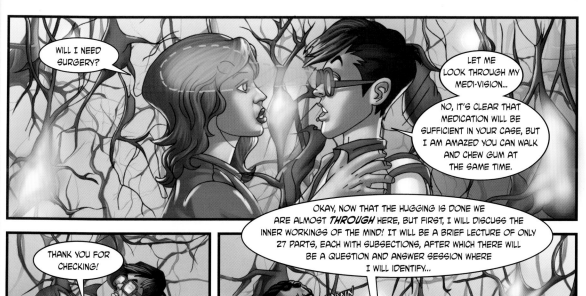

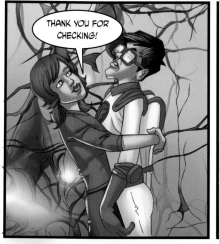

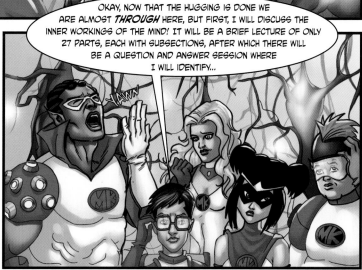

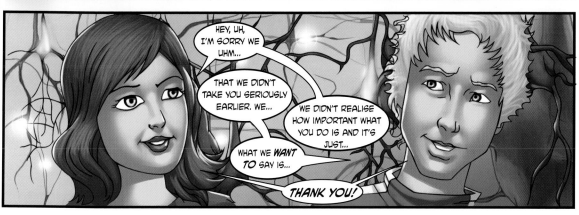

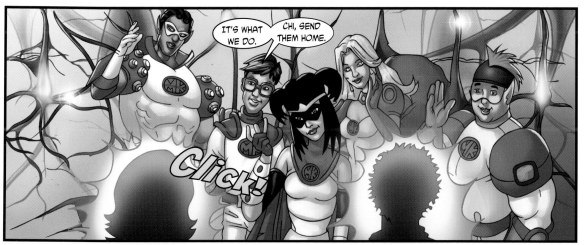

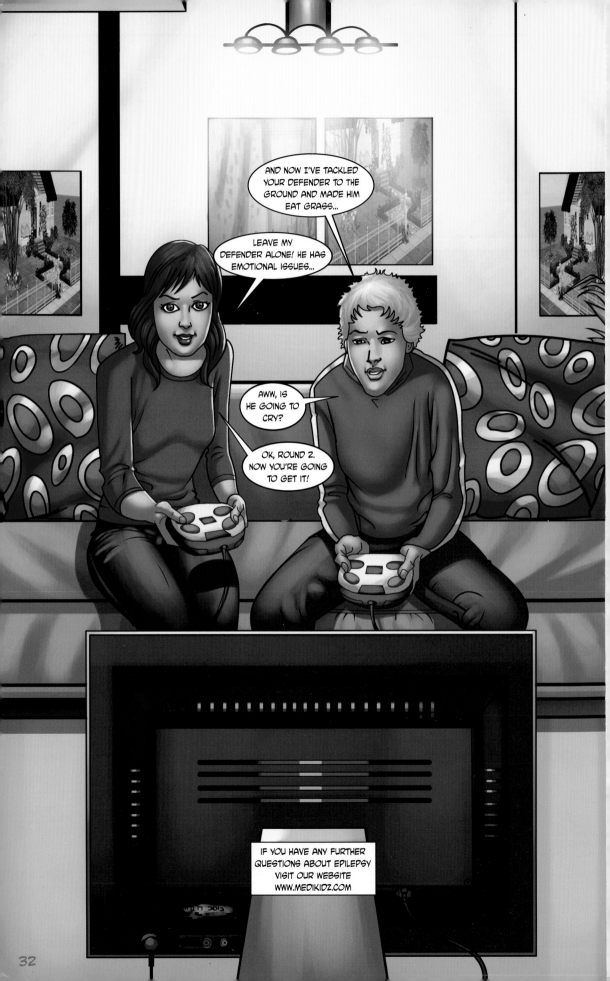